QUIT SMOKING

How to Master Your Life, Escape Nicotine Addiction With Results That Last

(How to Stop Smoking Now, Naturally, With or Without Hypnosis)

Crystal Peeples

Published by Harry Barnes

Crystal Peeples

All Rights Reserved

Quit Smoking: How to Master Your Life, Escape Nicotine Addiction With Results That Last (How to Stop Smoking Now, Naturally, With or Without Hypnosis)

ISBN 978-1-77485-103-6

All rights reserved. No part of this guide may be reproduced in any form without permission in writing from the publisher except in the case of brief quotations embodied in critical articles or reviews.

Legal & Disclaimer

The information contained in this book is not designed to replace or take the place of any form of medicine or professional medical advice. The information in this book has been provided for educational and entertainment purposes only.

The information contained in this book has been compiled from sources deemed reliable, and it is accurate to the best of the Author's knowledge; however, the Author cannot guarantee its accuracy and validity and cannot be held liable for any errors or omissions. Changes are periodically made to this book. You must consult your doctor or get professional medical advice before using any of the suggested remedies, techniques, or information in this book.

Upon using the information contained in this book, you agree to hold harmless the Author from and against any damages, costs, and expenses, including any legal fees potentially resulting from the application of any of the information provided by this guide. This disclaimer applies to any damages or injury caused by the use and application, whether directly or indirectly, of any advice or information presented, whether for breach of contract, tort, negligence, personal injury, criminal intent, or under any other cause of action.

You agree to accept all risks of using the information presented inside this book. You need to consult a professional medical practitioner in order to ensure you are both able and healthy enough to participate in this program.

Table of Contents

Introduction 1

Chapter 1: Effects Of Smoking 3

Chapter 2: Smokers' Behavior And Ideas . 7

Chapter 3: Digestion Side Effects 13

Chapter 4: A Sober Mind Does Not Assault Its Host... 31

Chapter 5: What Is Addiction? 40

Chapter 6: Understanding The Psychology Of Smoking 44

Chapter 7: Benefits Of Quit Smoking 64

Chapter 8: The First Time 70

Chapter 9: Marijuana Dependence 81

Chapter 10: Horrors Packed In A Stick Of Cigarette 86

Chapter 11: Smoking From A Psychological Perspective 97

Chapter 12: Understanding The Smoking Process 133

Chapter 13: Symptoms Of Nicotine Withdrawal 136

Chapter 14: Self-Hypnosis 141

Chapter 15: Smoke As Component Of Religious Beliefs 147

Chapter 16: Withdrawal Symptoms (How To Deal With Them) 154

Chapter 17: Plan You Put Down Personally To Stop The Habit Of Smoking 163

Chapter 18: Health 165

Conclusion 181

Introduction

Welcome!

I am truly happy and excited for you that you found this book and made the decision to read it because this itself implies that you really want to make a change and quit smoking for sure. I assume that you already tried to stop – possibly even multiple times before – but still ended up going back to it.

This book provides you with all the tools, strategies, and information you need in order to finally stop smoking and kick this habit for good. It will prepare and guide you through the process so you can live the way it is meant to be lived – smoke-free. All you need to do is to follow this proven success formula.

There are so many great benefits to quitting, so much to gain when you become smoke-free again but also so much to lose if you continue on that path. Above all, what you will get is more life, more strength, more happiness, more joy. On top of that, by quitting you will learn something that no non-smoker will ever have the chance to learn, which is true will power and the ability to overcome something as difficult as an addiction. This will make you a stronger individual that takes charge of life.

I know you are ready because you are sick and tired of this addiction having a hold on and controlling you. You don't have to be a slave any longer, you can be free, enjoy life again, and take deep breaths of fresh air. Many before you have quit, which means that you can do it too. It is possible. You can do this! We can do this!

Chapter 1: Effects Of Smoking

The primary bad outcomes of smoking are damage to your body, heavy financial cost, and the effects of secondhand smoking on your loved ones.

The damage to the body includes increased chance of cancer, heart disease and stroke, diabetes, cataracts, tooth loss, arthritis, infertility, and erectile dysfunction. Some of these illnesses may seem implausible, and a smoker may be wondering "erectile dysfunction? That can't be true." If you are looking for confirmation and need to do any further research, please check out the following link to the U.S. government website.

How cigarette smoking affects your body's internal organs is the most important reason to quit, but it also affects the skin.

Those who smoke look significantly older than their actual age. If you want to see how smoking affects the skin around your facial muscles, go to the following webmd link:

Pictures of identical twins are shown. The twin who smokes looks significantly older.

Another bad effect of smoking is financial. A pack of cigarettes costs about $4.00. If you have a half-a-pack-a-day smoking habit, this converts over a period of forty years to roughly a million dollars. Most people who quit smoking boast that the money spent on cigarettes now goes directly to their savings account or to buy fun things, such as motorcycles.

Another bad effect is secondhand smoke. A smoker causes serious health issues for all nonsmokers who live with them. According to the U.S. surgeon general, 2,500,000 nonsmoking adults have died because of secondhand smoke since 1964. Secondhand smoke causes significant damage to young children, increasing their chance of developing such respiratory illnesses as asthma. For adults, the risk of heart disease and lung cancer increases.

What's particularly astonishing about this statistic is that it was compiled by the U.S. government. America has just 5 percent of the world's population, but other parts of the world have similar smoking rates. There are roughly 1.2 billion smokers in the world, and smoking is the leading preventable cause of death worldwide. Globally, smoking has killed a hundred million people in the twentieth century, much more than all the deaths in two world wars. According to World Health Organization (WHO) experts, smoking-related deaths will number around one billion in the twenty-first century if current smoking patterns continue. The WHO and health ministries of all countries have smoking eradication as their top priority.

What's great, though, is that once you stop smoking your body quickly repairs itself. Your chance of stroke decreases by 50 percent within a year after you quit smoking. Within five to ten years, most ex-smokers have health outcomes similar to people who have never smoked. The following website provides a timetable that indicates the health benefits of quitting:

Chapter 2: Smokers' Behavior And Ideas

The desire for a cigarette is a very strange thing to try and explain to a non-smoker. Those who have never been addicted to nicotine must find it absolutely bizarre that an individual would choose to put a poisonous stick into their mouths and then set fire to it, repeatedly puff on it, knowing the damage they are doing to themselves and creating the most hideous smell in the process. Only a smoker or an ex-smoker can possibly understand it.

Smokers have very strange ideas about cigarettes and what they can achieve. Smokers believe that cigarettes enhance good times, cure boredom, lessen anxiety and relieve stress. When you think about it, how can they possibly do all of these things? The answer is, of course they can't, yet they are used by smokers as a kind of mental crutch. Allen Carr, the great anti-smoking

guru, who wrote incredibly readable books on how to give up smoking, wrote very compellingly on how smokers perceive cigarettes to be the perfect accompaniment to almost any kind of life situation. Cigarettes do not at all enhance good times. If anything, they diminish good times, as unless you are in the company only of smokers, and have the unrestricted ability to smoke, most smokers have to excuse themselves to go and smoke outside. How can a cigarette possibly relieve boredom? The answer is that it can't: a person who is bored who lights up a cigarette is still bored, but has the illusion that they are "doing something". What they are "doing", is damaging their health! Allen Carr wrote persuasively on how cigarettes are used by smokers in almost every situation that life could throw at them. They persuade themselves that cigarettes have this magical power, yet, in actual fact, all the smoker is doing is finding an excuse to get their next nicotine hit. Allen Carr was the first person who had ever written a book on smoking that really resonated with me. He invested the method he termed "the Easyway', which according to him, required no willpower, only the commonsense realisation that cigarettes were the cause of stress and not the remedy for stress. Very ironically, he died of lung cancer twenty-four years after he quit smoking, mainly because after he quit, he dedicated his life towards helping others to give up the habit, and spent many hours in the company of smokers. It was thought that exposure to passive smoking largely contributed towards his cancer.

I referred earlier to the psychological aspect of smoking addiction. There is an incredibly insidious aspect to tobacco addiction, and that is its social side. Smokers regard themselves as part of a club, a persecuted minority. There is a kind of shorthand amongst smokers, a kind of instant recognition, which when put in context is entirely understandable; they are nagged to death by their families, disapproved of by their non-smoking friends and colleagues, by institutions and organisations, many of which have banned smoking, and frown on its individual and societal effects. Therefore, when one smoker meets another, a kind of instant bond is formed. I have heard more than one person, my brother included, say that they have never met more interesting people than the ones they met when smoking. If you are smoking outside in a howling gail, freezing and risking a soaking just in order to get a nicotine fix, and someone is out there doing the same, inevitably, you will strike up a conversation with that person, even if they are a complete stranger. Go to any pub, and you will find a band of people outside smoking. Many of them, if stripped of their cigarettes would have absolutely nothing in common, but the little white sticks have given them a kind of badge, a membership to a club that requires a state of mind to belong. The same is true of office buildings. I used to work in the Tower 42 on Bishopsgate in the City of London, formerly known as the NatWest Tower. I had to descend 37 floors to exit the building in order to smoke. I struck up conversations with fellow smokers who worked in the building, many of whom worked in completely different industries, but who became familiar to me thanks to our shared habit.

In the 1970s, when my father was a young man, he went for a job interview. The person who was supposed to conduct the interview was absent that day, and therefore, my father was called in to a large office with a busy and distracted man who had not only one cigarette in his hand, but he also had several others 'on the go' in various ashtrays dotted around his office. Suddenly, in the middle of the interview, he stopped speaking abruptly, and was visibly horrified as he had run out of cigarettes. My father offered him one of his own cigarettes, a little known brand named Perilly's. They came in a black box, and were advertised as being 'slightly superior'. His interviewer was visibly relieved that a supply of cigarettes was available, and was noticeably surprised that my father smoked the same brand. My father is convinced to this day that he was offered the job for this reason, and that reason alone.

Chapter 3: Digestion Side Effects

Symptoms • Duration • Treatment

Nausea

This symptom almost seems like the flu. The duration typically lasts about a week. The treatment would be to drink lots of water and a carbonated beverage—which should help.

"For the first 3 days I had headaches, nausea and diarrhea."

—Karen

"I've quit smoking (cold turkey) for more than 2 months. I smoked eighteen years. Now I am feeling dizziness, headache, vomiting, and body and muscle pain."

—Aman

Diarrhea

This symptom typically can last a few days. Try any over-the-counter remedy for diarrhea. The body is adjusting to the new digestive changes.

"I smoked for 17 years at a rate of 12-15 cigarettes per day. Four months back I stopped smoking cold turkey. Needless to say I have suffered enormously due to the lack of knowledge of the impact of cold turkey. My pains started 3 days after stopping. The inner lining of my mouth was sore. I had severe stomach problems (bloating, cramps lasting up to 8 weeks), diarrhea for a day, inability to hold onto food. The more I stressed about my symptoms, the worse my stomach problems got."

—Hishy

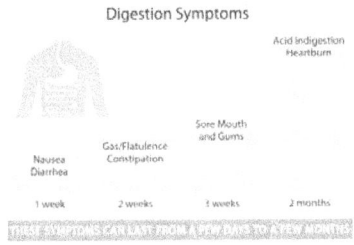

Gas or Flatulence

Try to avoid eating gas-producing foods like beans, cabbage, or cauliflower. This symptom can last for several weeks.

Try Beano to relieve the symptoms of gas.

"I smoked 2 packs a day for 25 years and quit smoking cold turkey 3 weeks ago. Anyway, from my list of torments in the past 24 days: Enormous quantity of gas in my body (I have a slim/athletic build and I never had this problem before.) It's quite embarrassing because the smell is unbearable and it's not related to food."

—MickeyNBG

Constipation

This may last several weeks. Cigarettes act like a diuretic and also a laxative in the body so when you take nicotine away you can get constipated. You can use an over-the-counter remedy or make your own homemade laxative recipe that is natural and gentler on the body.

"Since I quit smoking cold turkey I have been dealing with bloating, fluid retention and strange pains in my intestines and gut. I have had heartburn all the time and a strange pain in my throat that comes and goes (sometimes, I can feel it up into my bottom teeth.)"

—Jenn L.

"I quit smoking about 9 weeks ago and at first, it was OK. After about 4 -5 weeks, I became so incredibly constipated that I believed I had rectal/bowel cancer. I have had a pelvic ultrasound and numerous x-rays because I am so *convinced* I am dying. I have been trying to drink extra water and add fiber to my diet, but, I have also been suffering from heartburn and indigestion. I am still suffering from all three of these *ailments.*"

—jlove418

Homemade Laxative Recipe

Ingredients	Instructions
8 oz. dried prunes 8 oz. raisins 8 oz. dried figs 2 oz. Senna tea leaves crushed or buy Senna tea bags and open up some bags (Senna leaves may be hard to find.) ¼ C lemon juice 2½ C water ¼ C brown sugar ½ C prune juice	Bring prunes, raisins, figs, Senna leaves, lemon juice and water to a boil. Boil for 15 to 20 minutes. Remove from heat and add brown sugar. Allow to cool. Using a mixer, turn into a smooth paste while gradually adding prune juice. Put in several plastic containers with lids

	and store in freezer. It will be the consistency of ice cream. Take 1 tablespoon every morning and evening day (Use it as a spread.)

Note–This recipe can be printed out from our website. www.nicotinesolutions.com/homemade-laxative-recipe/

Quit Smoking Side Effects Timetable

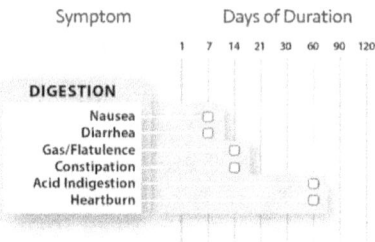

Alkaline/Acidic Foods

If you are still on any form of nicotine replacement therapy (NRT) like the nicotine patch, gum, lozenge or e-cigarette, then you are not detoxifying from nicotine. When you smoked, your body used nicotine as a laxative or it was an "aid in digestion" so you are not out of the woods until you are completely off of the nicotine in any form.

What you are doing with the patch is giving your body nicotine with a different delivery system. I am not taking away anything from your accomplishment; I am just saying that you will still have to detoxify from nicotine when you stop using the patch.

Acid indigestion is aggravated by acidic foods. Try to avoid eating these. Eat highly alkaline-based foods to help with digestion. Here is a list of highly alkaline foods that will help:

Highly Alkaline Foods

Almond Milk

Artichokes

Arugula

Asparagus

Avocado

Baby Potatoes

Beans & Legumes

Broccoli

Brussels Sprouts

Butter beans

Cabbage

Carrot

Cauliflower

Celery

Chives

Coconut

Collard

Cucumber

Endive

Garlic

Ginger

Goat's Milk

Grapefruit

Green Beans

Kale

Kelp

Leeks

Lemon

Lentils

Lettuce

Lime

Mustard Greens

Okra

Onion

Parsley

Peas

Quinoa

Radish

Red Onion

Soy Beans

Spinach

Sprouted Beans (all)

Tomato

Watercress

Zucchini

If you have heartburn or acid indigestion avoid eating the following highly acidic foods:

Highly Acidic Foods

Alcohol

Artificial Sweetener

Beef

Black Tea

Cheese

Chicken

Cocoa

Coffee

Dairy

Dried Fruit

Eggs

Fish

Jam

Jelly

Mushrooms

Pork

Shellfish

Soy Sauce

Sugar

Syrup

Vinegar

Yeast

Stomach Pain

This is due to a change in how the body processes food. It should only last a week or two.

Jenn L. to Robin J.,

"Since quitting smoking, I have had a pelvic ultrasound for lower abdominal pain and leg pain; I have had several chest x-rays for bone abnormalities and possible tumors. The only thing the x-rays showed were arthritis of the middle back, a curvature of the spine and issues with my neck. I have had two CBC's run and some other blood work done. (Editor's note: CBC stands for complete blood count).I have been to so many doctors since I quit to the point where I think most of them think I am crazy. I seem to be having all of the symptoms listed, but they are staggered."

—Jenn L.

"I stopped smoking 6 weeks ago by going cold turkey. This is the first time I have quit smoking and am so proud of myself, but I have suffered badly. I had palpitations, even went to the hospital on an EKG machine, all ok. Had all my blood tests done—all ok too. Felt so emotional at times, cried for no reason, tingles in my left arm, still have dizziness but not as bad as when I first quit. I'm now suffering with constipation and acid indigestion."

—Emma

Over the years I have discovered many over-the-counter remedies for the side effects of quitting smoking.

Throughout the book I recommended different products that have been proven to relieve side effects and symptoms. I have combined 6 of them into a *Kick Butt Recovery Kit* that you can read about in the back of the book.

In this chapter on digestion I recommend Tums (an antacid) and Beano to help with flatulence or gas.

Chapter 4: A Sober Mind Does Not Assault Its Host

Yes, it's true that many people turn to expensive counseling, buying nicotine patches, or to pursuing other costly methods for getting themselves to quit smoking.

But in order for you to be fully conscious, you must remain sober at all times, as this is the only way we humans can have proper judgment at all levels of our reasoning about the things we think and do. Having control over your behavior is crucial to the way you live, and that means your mind must be sober.

A BREACH OF SOBRIETY was what started your smoking, so that breach must be reversed in order for you to regain full control of yourself.

If I ask you whether or not it was a good idea to START smoking, logically you would say no; and if I ask what caused you to start smoking, you will find that your mind was not thinking correctly at the time. Perhaps it was peer pressure, or the portrayal of smoking as cool or debonair. Maybe your parents or guardians smoked like chimneys.

Any time we neglect to think properly, we leave ourselves wide open for attack by negative situations. This means that we must train ourselves to have a one hundred percent (100%) unbroken consciousness for maintaining full accountability of our behavior.

No person who retains sobriety ever becomes a smoker, because good judgment and accurate distinction do not allow a deliberate evil to prevail in his or her system.

The key to avoiding the voluntary defilement of your body is to work so that your mind will always reason coherently as it relates to your own well being.

Do you think the emphysema patient thought he was choosing to destroy his body's ability to breathe when he became a smoker? Or that the woman with a mouth full of painful malignant ulcers thought she was assaulting her mouth every. single. time. she lit one up?

No. But they certainly displayed a callous disregard for their vehicle through life – their bodies – the second they held the first cigarette to their lips. But naturally, the mind wasn't looking at it that way.

The human body (including yours) is primarily governed by the <u>subconscious</u> mind, and our secondary <u>conscious</u> mind works in partnership with our subconscious mind on issues pertaining to bodily function. Having said that, here is a very important fact, something many smokers who have tried to quit do not realize, which ultimately causes them to fail — they are using solutions that circumvent the mind's administrative process.

Yet logic shows that it was a mental decision that prompted you to start smoking. So how logical is it to attempt to solve the problem with any method that doesn't take your attention into your mind?

There is a natural and intelligent way to correct the addiction of smoking, and you as the commander of your mind need not be relegated to endless trial and error — which is essentially AN ABUSE OF YOUR BIOLOGICAL SYSTEM.

Cancer and emphysema aside, the foreign substances of cigarettes inhibit the production of the healthy hormones that support you in being a well-balanced and civilized individual. *This is what makes it so hard to get help from your body and mind to quit.* You've essentially chased out the healthy agents and replaced them with destructive ones.

Before we get to the panacea, let us first take a walk through some of the methods that are most commonly used to quit smoking.

The following methods are used by millions of people to give up their cigarettes every day. This confirms that there is not just one way to attempt to stop smoking, but many ex-smokers will tell you that there is one common truth...

<u>You always want to quit!</u>

The Most Common Ways to Stop Smoking:

1. Quitting 'cold turkey' or just stopping

2. Prescription medication or pills

3. Nicotine replacement therapy (NRT)

4. Zyban tablets

5. Taper down method or gradual phase out

6. Hypnosis

7. Acupuncture

8. Laser therapy

9. Chantix program

10. Counseling or therapy, vapor, etc.

We see all the different methods that people implement, trying ever so hard to overcome their cigarette smoking addition. And you should agree that the fact that people are willing to try these things proves they are quite undisciplined in their thinking and, as such, have very little control of their thoughts.

But it is important to invest the time it takes to gain control of the way you think, as quantum physics has shown that **thoughts are creative**. So if you continue to believe in your body's addiction, you will continue to experience great struggle in overcoming it.

So let's look briefly at the psychology at work here. You got caught up in a careless habit, and continued to do it until you developed a serious addiction. Even though you may have seen people walking around with oxygen tanks and tubes up their noses to help them breathe. And even though you'd no doubt heard reports of people dying from smoking-related illnesses and diseases, you still neglected to make attempts to stop with the smoking.

For maybe one, five, ten, fifteen, or even twenty years, you purchased cigarettes like you were buying food, some of you unable to even wait for the 10:30 AM break to leave your workplace for a cigarette.

People define mental strength in many different ways. For some people, as long as one can drive from home to work, you are mentally sound. However, this is not true, as to function effectively consciousness must be balanced.

This is also the key to overcoming the symptoms of withdrawal from the body's addiction to nicotine, and subsequent cravings to replace smoking with other ill-conceived habits.

The mind is a very delicate yet powerful entity, and people who don't understand how simultaneously fragile and powerful it is, are almost certain to experience great disaster in their lives.

Chapter 5: What Is Addiction?

Addiction in a broader sense defines the repetition of a specific behaviour even if that behaviour has negative consequences. To be more specific, drug addiction defines the continual compulsive use of one or multiple drugs even when the use of those drugs is causing harm. Drug addiction is often associated with a development of tolerance to the specific drug, withdrawal symptoms on discontinuation, and significant adverse consequences. Addiction is multifactorial, and this is why it is often so hard to break.

Nicotine is a great example of a drug which causes harm to the user, unpleasant withdrawal symptoms on discontinuation and tolerance. When nicotine is inhaled, it floods into the brain and binds to receptors in the brain known as nicotinic receptors. Once nicotine binds to these receptors, a complex series of messages are processed in the brain and ultimately the brain releases a neurotransmitter known as dopamine.

Dopamine is responsible for what is known as reward-motivated behaviour. When you do something that increases dopamine in your central nervous system, you will feel good and feel motivated to do it again. This urges the user to continue smoking to receive continual surges of dopamine. It is now understood that dopamine levels in the central nervous system also surge when the brain is exposed to other addictive drugs such as cocaine and amphetamines.

Of course, the dopamine reward system is only part of the reason why people become addicted to nicotine. Many people continue to smoke tobacco to avoid withdrawal symptoms. Withdrawal symptoms from nicotine can include irritability, difficulty concentrating, restlessness, cravings and appetite changes. Others may find it hard quitting because they find the whole process of smoking tobacco addictive and with years of use it can become ingrained into their lives. Rolling the tobacco, lighting up, bringing the cigarette to their mouth and inhaling can be quiet an addictive process. Other people may continue to go places or do things that they associated with smoking, such as smoking on their work break or going to the pub. Of course, some people continue smoking because they simply don't want to quit.

Nicotine results in a rapid onset of addiction; cravings may develop within days of starting tobacco smoking. A psychological and physical dependence to nicotine can develop within a couple of weeks of constant use. Psychological dependence is when someone feels the urge to use a substance to affect their mood or prevent the possibility of withdrawal symptoms. A physical dependence to a substance occurs when withdrawal symptoms occur in the absence of that substance. The majority of tobacco smokers will have both a psychological and physical dependence to nicotine.

Chapter 6: Understanding The Psychology Of Smoking

Two or three years back, everybody thought it was cool to smoke in broad daylight. A few people even suggested that smoking helped you get an edge on your companions by giving you a demeanor of certainty when puffing ceaselessly. With a cigarette you were the one everybody needed to resemble in your friend network. It was accepted that the other gender was evidently more pulled in to you, in the event that you were elegantly smoking endlessly. Smoking is accepted by some to make the man more virile.

Despite the fact that you may ask why everything that is seen as cool is connected with virility, how about we center around this entire cigarette business and how it has for all intents and purposes pushed humanity to the brink of collapse. An all around led overview factually uncovers realities about smoking and its destructive impacts on the body. The investigation thought about the effect of the harm making passings smokers like the annihilation of the individuals who kicked the bucket in the Hiroshima and Nagasaki bombings in Japan.

At the present time, researchers name smoking as the biggest preventable reason for untimely sicknesses and early passing. Consistently, one of every fifteen grown-ups is kicking the bucket of lung disease. This is credited to the addictive idea of smoking, bringing about a yearly 4,000,000 passings (this is a surmised figure). Tobacco utilization relates to smoking, yet in addition biting betel leaves and breathing in destructive snuff. Yet at the same time notwithstanding these realities it merits seeing that roughly 15 billion cigarettes are sold day by day. That is a HUGE figure! Who smokes that much and WHY?

Around one out of three cigarettes devoured is in the Western Pacific Region of the world. The tobacco advertise is constrained by only a couple of enterprises - to be specific American, British and Japanese global combinations. Among youthful youngsters (matured 13 - 15), around one of every five smokes all through the world. They enjoy this barbarous propensity known as "fagging" in spite of monitoring the way that tobacco smoke contains in excess of 4,000 cancer-causing substances. At the point when a smoker smokes within the sight of non smokers, he is influencing them with poisonous substances, maybe more than himself. It has been demonstrated experimentally that uninvolved smoking has been seen as the most exceedingly terrible and most flighty reason for monstrous sicknesses on different populaces.

Around 80,000 to 100,000 youngsters begin smoking each day. These figures incorporate the two young people and adolescents. There is a propensity for the individuals who begin to smoke at a youthful age to not have the option to stop in their adulthoods. What pushes these young people to carelessly follow a prevailing fashion which later proceeds to get one of their life's most concerning issues? Maybe it's the marvelous promotions of cigarettes, where the smoker is demonstrated to be the alpha male. Where the "genuine man" is equipped for accomplishing the most unimaginable of accomplishments against the most far-fetched of chances since he smokes. On the off chance that it isn't so much that it just might be their top choice celebrities illuminating in style, not long before a serious snapshot of activity or a strategic maneuver. What youngster wouldn't have any desire to emulate that picture? Analysts inferred that all the up to referenced factors certainly stirs an individual's craving to smoke. In any case, in the event that we truly need to get to the base of this puzzle, we should begin at the very underlying foundations of the issue. We have to invest significant time to comprehend the brain science of smoking and why it's so difficult to surrender the irresistible propensity.

At whatever point researchers begin breaking down any issue, they first search for the indications of the ailment. It is sheltered to state the smoking is an ailment of dependence. In the event that you have been dependent on cigarettes for a satisfactory piece of your life, you would have seen that the hardest piece of stopping is to beat the yearnings. A vigorously reliant smoker needs only one more cigarette pretty much every other moment of his waking hours. Indeed, even in his rest he has smoke-murky fantasies about getting a charge out of outlandish forms of cigarettes. Addicts report that after a state of time, the smoking propensity dominates so seriously and unwittingly that one beginnings smoking regardless of where he is, or what he is doing. Following a day of difficult work, so as to loosen up an individual may want to smoke till he gets distinctly languid. It is nicotine, the dynamic and the most destructive synapse present in tobacco that effectively numbs his detects.

Knopfler may have celebrated the way that demigods have nicotine for breakfast, however Angus legitimately said that 'smoking turns one too old to even think about rocking and roll yet too youthful to even consider dieing!' How is it that nicotine effectively assumes control over the human brain and causes us to lose control of our bodies and lives?

Acetylcholine is one of the most significant neurotransmitters present in the body. Acetylcholine nerve receptors at the neural connections take after those of nicotine. Nicotine hurries to the torment receptors and other sense receptors and hinders these destinations stopping the ordinary section of apprehensive drive. This causes the blockage of data fundamental for the focal sensory system to work so as the outcome transmitters continue attempting to arrive at the essential pathways. For some odd reason with each extra cigarette the impact gets increasingly articulated. When you are finished with your first puff, the impression of deadness wears off quick and so as to draw out the fluffy inclination, you unwittingly connect for another cigarette. This is one of the essential side effects of nicotine instigated withdrawals, something which is the very germ of the entire smoking disaster. Recollect that each cigarette cleared removes in any event five minutes of your typical life expectancy. Is that a cheerful idea? Consider it!

Each cigarette maker gives the disclaimer on their pack of cigarettes that "Cigarette smoking is harmful to wellbeing." Now this may appear to be a trick, very nearly a test to your safe framework, however the Physician General who composes the disclaimer does so in light of the fact that he has seen the expansive outcomes of nicotine, similar to lung malignant growth and unexpected passing.

Have you known about the Pavlovian investigation? The renowned Russian scholar found that he can cause a canine to salivate during its eating time without really serving him food. He did as such by ringing a bell which set off a drive of longing for in its sensory system. So also in a smoker, it is discovered that in the event that they are familiar with smoking in nearness of some espresso or in the organization of companions, their body is adapted to needing to smoke close to such improvements.

The Smokers Quiz

Is it accurate to say that you are Addicted To Smoking?

How on earth did you get dependent on smoking? You may have been pondering this for some time without having any piece of information about it. Through this part, we will attempt to assist you with deciding if you're really dependent on smoking or not.

Recall the first occasion when you smoked?

A great many people recount to a comparable anecdote about their first cigarette. It goes this way: You were spending time with a couple of companions, one of them gave you a cigarette and requested that you perceive how it felt to take a drag. You attempted to breathe in it, hacked over it and there....that was your first smoke.

For what reason did you proceed at any rate? Like the others, did you see the propensity for smoking as a pressure remover? Did you want to rely upon smoking to take your concerns and the weakness away? Does it mitigate you, and satisfy you?

Somehow, cigarettes have ended up being the cool way out, particularly among youths. Your body may abhor it, however your psyche is continually impelling you to go on in case you begin passing up something.

Obviously once you are all into it, smoking resembles a prop that you need so you can keep strolling in your life. You spend heaps of cash on it; you limit your life expectancy but then you continue endlessly. You believe it's the tricky enhancement to life that props you up. Try not to be distraught about your reasons in light of the fact that these are similar reasons that a large number of different smokers use as well.

You may have attempted to stop, however it is truly not as simple as you suspected. You might be stressed over the withdrawal indications that you may need to manage, in addition to other things. Some way or another the entire recommendation of stopping smoking appears to be excessively ridiculous for you.

Here, as we let you assess your habit and the potential qualities related with it, you will scarcely believe, it isn't about just responding to a couple of inquiries. It is likewise about letting you decide for yourself what the issues are and how much your reliance on cigarettes is.

It is up to you presently to choose whether you need to wriggle liberated from the propensity or simply surrender to your fixation and let it keep on controlling your life.

Investigate these inquiries:

1. Do you smoke day by day? In the event that so for how long have you been smoking day by day?

2. Check the accompanying rundown and answer genuinely to yourself, which of these do you experience after you stop or cut down on the measure of smoking. These indications can set in following you have taken a break from smoking.

Nervousness

Diminishing in pulse

Misery and emotional episodes

Trouble in concentrating

Expanded hunger or weight gain

A sleeping disorder

Anxiety

Unexplainable touchiness, disappointment or outrage

3. How severely do the side effects referenced above set in when you experience them? Do you need to defer all work as a result of them?

Check if the response to all or the majority of the indications above is yes. In the event that it is an indeed, it's the ideal opportunity for you to get some assistance. Make an effort not to linger now since you are beginning to see that your enslavement is more awful than you at first idea. Rather than being trying to claim ignorance; spare that vitality to get together all the mental fortitude you have to take on this issue head-on.

4. Would you be able to recall a solitary day in the most recent year or so when you didn't smoke by any means?

In the event that you can recollect a day in your life where you didn't smoke at that point, attempt to recall how you figured out how to remain liberated from smoking that day. Attempt and re-institute very similar things you did that day that shielded you from smoking. In the event that you can't recall not smoking, at that point don't stress, you're not alone. It doesn't mean you should surrender all together on stopping. It's simply implies you have to invest more energy into your next endeavor. It's not the apocalypse, simply include a little tolerance and quality of psyche to the condition and before you know it you will be liberated from cigarettes for good.

5. Do you smoke despite having a condition identified with tobacco

dependence like bronchitis or COPD (Chronic Obstructive Pulmonary Disease)?

In the event that you are encountering any diseases identified with smoking, at that point recall that most smokers do have a feeling of the clinical issues that they face from their propensity. A lung condition, a heart condition, a mouth condition, or general reactions doesn't stop the dependent smoker. Nothing discourages them since they are dependent on the nicotine regardless of the negative wellbeing impacts that they might be encountering while they keep on smoking.

6. Is the delight or fulfillment from smoking turning out to be less consistently?

Smokers will in general find that so as to get a similar inclination that they used to get from their cigarettes when they started smoking, that they need increasingly more to make up for that feeling.

7. Do you smoke as much consistently notwithstanding noting yes to the above inquiry?

As a result of the ongoing media presentation a great deal of smokers are getting a reminder. The dangers of malignant growth and ailments are very genuine yet the fiend knows this yet essentially can't stop. In the event that you keep on smoking, in spite of monitoring all its negative impacts then clearly you have an issue. For what other reason would you readily expose your body to harm?

8. Is it true that you are as yet a major fanatic of cigarettes in spite of knowing about all the negative wellbeing impacts?

On the off chance that you said truly, at that point go over the realities about smoking in your mind by and by. It murders at long last. It eases back down your reflexes and you are actually harming your body. It doesn't benefit you in any way. It is simply in your mind and has a power over you. You are not dependent by decision. Your brain and body both long for nicotine, however the compulsion isn't difficult to break. It resembles you are under a spell. You need to stop yet you feel constrained to have one more cigarette. It might sound excess, yet the more you disguise these announcements, the quicker you are to break free.

9. Have you been on edge or anxious for the initial fourteen days of stopping smoking at whatever point you have attempted?

In the event that indeed, at that point unmistakably these are a piece of your withdrawal side effects. Try not to stress. This doesn't imply that you don't have it in you to stop smoking. It just implies that you need to rouse yourself somewhat more. You need to battle somewhat harder with your psyche. You need somewhat more solidarity to proceed and we will assist you with working up the inward solidarity to defeat the propensity.

10. Have you been discouraged for the initial fourteen days after you have attempted to stopped smoking?

On the off chance that your answer is indeed, at that point by and by we rehash, it isn't the greatest snag. Again you have to approach your inward quality. Work on your trust in your choice to stop and endure each hour in turn. Recollect the mantra-"It isn't hard to stop." You simply need to manage it in your mind.

Chapter 7: Benefits Of Quit Smoking

According to estimates, around 110,000 people die in around the globe every year from the consequences of tobacco and cigarette consumption. Smoking is the most significant risk factor for lung cancer and favours many other cancers. In addition, smoking increases the risk of having a stroke or heart attack and developing visual disturbances, poor circulation, asthma or other lung diseases. Overall, smoking weakens the immune system and can adversely affect the course of many other diseases. Smoking cessation, therefore, always has a positive effect on health, regardless of how long and how much has been smoked before.

How does smoking cessation affect the body?

Nicotine affects the human body and psyche in a variety of ways. Some of the effects show up immediately, and others increase over the years. However, the first positive effects of stopping smoking can be seen after a very short time. Immediately after the last cigarette, the body begins to recover and reverse the harmful effects of nicotine consumption.

Blood pressure normalizes on the 1st day after the last cigarette

Nicotine constricts the blood vessels, speeds up the heartbeat and increases the amount of blood pumped from the heart and consequently the blood pressure. About 20 minutes after the last smoked cigarette, heartbeat and blood pressure normalize again.

Smoking gets carbon monoxide (CO) into the body and blocks about 10 percent of red blood cells there. The level of CO in the body only drops again about 8 to 12 hours after smoking. This has the positive consequence that more red blood cells can transport oxygen into the tissues and organs, which they urgently need for their work. Physical performance increases due to the better oxygen supply. Those who survived the first day without cigarettes have already slightly reduced their risk of a heart attack.

After 2 days, the nerve endings regenerate

After two days without nicotine, the nerve endings begin to regenerate. The taste and smell become more intense; the perception of individual aromas becomes easier. Many former smokers report that at this stage, they have noticed certain smells, such as field and meadow flowers, for the first time in years.

The stuck mucus loosens 2 weeks after stopping smoking

After about two weeks, the blood circulation and lungs start to regenerate and continue for the next 3 months. Now that the mucus, which has been stuck in the air for some time, is now loosening, breathing becomes much easier. Lung function can increase by almost a third. Sufferers feel that they no longer get out of breath as quickly under physical strain.

After 9 to 12 months, the smoker's cough weakens

It takes about nine months for the so-called smoker's cough to weaken and the number of cough cases to decrease. The cilia in the bronchi have grown back and can work again unhindered. Your task is to transport dust and dirt particles in the airways out. Among other things, these are responsible for making smokers more susceptible to colds and other infections.

The risk of stroke drops 5 years after the last cigarette

According to German Stroke Help, the risk of suffering a stroke is twice as high for smokers as for non-smokers. However, about five years after the last cigarette, it has dropped significantly and can again be at the same level as a non-smoker.

The risk of cancer decreases after 10 years

After 10 years without nicotine, the cancer risk of former smokers decreases. This primarily affects air and esophageal cancer and oral cancer. The risk of lung cancer also decreases and is about half lower than in people who still smoke. In the meantime, cells that already had tissue changes have been broken down by the body and replaced by healthy new cells.

After 15 years, the body recovers from the effects of smoking

It takes almost 15 years to reduce the risk of cardiovascular disease to the level of a lifelong non-smoker. If smoking has not caused any permanent damage by then, the body has then recovered from the negative effects of smoking.

Chapter 8: The First Time

Just looking at what arrived from Newtons Traditional Remedies told me this was never going to work. Inside the padded envelope were two white plastic pots. The labels were simple black ink on white paper, and in one pot was "the smoking cure". These were small white tablets with a kind of greenish fleck in them, but unremarkable otherwise. The other pot's label was titled "nerve aid pills" to calm me while the smoking cure was doing its thing. The pills were sugar coated, like M&Ms. There were, if I remember correctly, 100 pills in each pot. Also included was a photocopied single sheet of paper. This flyer explained that the smoking cure was based on Lobelia, and it would completely remove the nicotine from my system as though I had never smoked. The instructions, such as they were, said I should suck a smoking cure tablet as often as I would smoke a cigarette. It was quite specific about that – don't just take them like a normal tablet with water, but instead dissolve them on your tongue.

Remember, this was back in the 80s, before we became such a risk-averse society, so there were no health warnings or disclaimers of liability or anything like that.

To my wife, I hid my total scepticism – after all, the amount I had paid would be an excellent investment if it stopped her asking me to stop smoking. I determined I would take the cure in a couple of days and give it my best shot. Not that it could possibly work.

At the time I was working as a business development manager for a transport company that sent trucks on long-distance runs all over Europe. It wasn't a difficult job. About 25% of it involved wining and dining potential new customers and existing key accounts. A real fun aspect of the job was that I could decide to take a truck out and drive around Europe when the mood took me. The business reason would be we needed some promotional photos of one of our trucks in, say Lisbon, Madrid, Monaco, Milan or Stockholm. Or, to impress someone at a company I was trying to develop as a customer, I would make a sales call somewhere in Europe, in one of our trucks. Of course, that meant I always got to play with the newest and best trucks in the fleet. It was a great job.

When I wasn't entertaining in restaurants and at major events, or swanning around Europe in a truck, it was a drive of over an hour each morning to get to the office, taking London's M25 motorway. I figured I would start the cure first thing one Monday morning, so instead of my first cigarette when I opened my eyes, I would take and suck a smoking cure tablet and get the process started.

I smoked right up to the time I went to sleep, and I deliberately didn't put my packet of cigarettes and lighter on the bedside table. I woke up and took the first pill and yuck! It tasted absolutely foul. I dissolved it on my tongue as the instructions said, and then I went and got a strong coffee to get rid of the taste.

I got in the car and headed to the office with my packet of cigarettes, which had about 16 left, and the lighter on the central console. I sucked a couple more smoking cure tablets on the journey to work, and, strangely, while they still tasted foul, I didn't have any cravings to smoke a cigarette. I did also try a couple of the nerve aid tablets, but I didn't see that they did anything for me.

At work, as the hours passed, I began to feel quite odd. I can't accurately describe it. But there was something not quite right. I felt confused, and my mood was blackening. It was as if someone had picked me up and shaken me vigorously so that my head was spinning, and my mind was taking its time to get itself back to normal. And, amazingly, though I had my cigarettes and lighter in my pocket and could have got one out and tried to smoke it, I just didn't have the inclination. I think that was partly influenced by the warning that during the course of the cure, cigarettes would taste pretty bad if one weakened. So it didn't occur to me to do that, and that was not because of any willpower. Something was happening, and I simply didn't think to smoke. That was pretty amazing since I had previously found it difficult to go two hours without smoking.

Driving back home from work, I tried to rationalise it or understand why I was feeling so odd. At the time, I had been smoking for close on 20 years. And not just smoking – chain smoking. If this Lobelia stuff was really doing what they said it would do and it was blasting away all that history as though I had never smoked in the first place, then clearly there was a huge battle going on inside me. Indeed, I have often said I don't smoke – I am a total nicotine addict. I really can't control it. And here I was – the nicotine replaced with the lobelia and it seemed to be working. I had, and still have, no idea how that works.

And still, I carried on taking the smoking cure tablets – I guess I had taken about a dozen since I woke up that morning when I arrived home 12 hours later. My wife was waiting at the door for me, all hopeful and asking, "How has it gone. Have you smoked …?"

"No," I cut her short, which was very uncharacteristic of me. "I feel odd. I'm going to bed."

When I said I felt odd, it wasn't an illness thing. I wasn't ill or nauseous or anything like that. I just felt odd inside, mainly in my head which clearly couldn't understand what was happening. And I knew I couldn't discuss it or chat about this smoking cure. So it was best I didn't try.

I didn't even bother with an evening meal and just went to bed by 7.30 pm. I slept right through until the following morning when the alarm went off. I awoke with an even blacker mood and still feeling shook up inside. I quickly packed an overnight bag and said to my wife, "I'm going to work and I'm going to take a truck out to

Europe today. This cure seems to be working, but I don't want to be around people. I'm in a peculiar mood."

I got to the office and commandeered the newest truck in the fleet that had only been delivered the day before. I told my boss I needed to get away for a couple of days and he was cool with that, so off I went with a load heading for northern Spain.

I was extremely grumpy on that second day of taking the tablets, with whatever they were doing to me. More than that, I would have loved to punch someone! So, being on my own in the cab of a truck heading down through France to near the Spanish border was the best place for me. I still had no desire to have a cigarette – yes, the packet and my lighter came with me – and sucking the tablets became less distasteful. I can't say I was growing to like them, but I knew what awfulness to expect.

I am perennially laid back and happy go lucky, but I was a now a very, very grumpy person. I didn't phone my wife to let her know how the trip was going or how I was – I felt sure I would snap at something in the conversation and I just didn't want to do that. Mostly, she would want to ask how the cure was going, and I just wasn't capable of discussing it.

On the fourth day, my mood was at its blackest, and I did wonder what I would be like the next day. And that was the astonishing part: I woke up my usual, joking, light-hearted self! It was as if someone had flicked a switch. Indeed, I found the first phone box (remember it was the days before the ubiquitous mobile phone) at a truck stop in France and called my wife. I was bubbling, glowing and happy, and apologised for being grumpy and not phoning her to let her know how I was getting on.

"But, have you smo….."

"Not a one. It's worked. I just don't have any desire to."

I had delivered the load I had taken and I just couldn't wait to get home to my wife. And it would be a new, non-smoking life.

Hold on! I can sense your confusion. Here I am, talking about how I took this miracle Lobelia cure that would blast the nicotine out of my system and leave me with a clean sheet as though I had never smoked. And now, 30 years later, I'm telling you that tomorrow I am about to take this miracle cure again. So, obviously, it doesn't actually work?

Yes it does. But let me tell you what went wrong — the thing I never anticipated or made allowances for.

And another point: if you are a chain-smoker who finds it hell to go without a cigarette for more than two hours, let alone an entire day, then something that stops you smoking, or having any desire to smoke, for even one week, is, in my book, a cure.

Chapter 9: Marijuana Dependence

People use marijuana to de-stress as it makes them feel like the time has slowed down, making them feel relaxed. Not everyone likes to mention the sickening feelings, the thumping heart, and the nausea. In the 5th revision of DSM-5 (Diagnostic and Statistical Manual of Mental Disorders), marijuana dependence is defined as a condition requiring treatment. At least 9% of the people who smoke marijuana become dependent on it. In America, between 10 and 20 percent of regular marijuana smokers become dependent on it.

Symptoms of Dependence

Of course, once you become dependent, there are symptoms that confirm the dependence. Following are some common symptoms of marijuana dependence:

People who are dependent on marijuana continue using this drug even when they know all its harmful effects.

They continue using marijuana even if it causes them health problems.

They miss out on the things that matter, skip school, work, jobs, and daily chores and choose to smoke up instead.

They spend most of their time looking for obtaining marijuana.

They spend most of their time abusing/using this drug.

They waste most of their time recovering from marijuana and its hangover.

Sometimes people realize that marijuana is not healthy and try to quit it, but end up breaking their resolve, because they are dependent on it.

Another sign of addiction and dependence is that the user plans and tries to smoke up less, either to quit or just reduce the amount smoked, but fails at it and ends up using more than intended.

They develop a tolerance for marijuana. In order to get high the way they want, they need to smoke more than the previous amount, and the amount they smoke up next time keeps increasing steadily

Withdrawal Symptoms

Anyone dependent on marijuana will also experience withdrawal symptoms if they stop using marijuana or do not use it for a period of time longer than they usually do. With time, the intervals decrease and the smoking up increases. The withdrawal symptoms include:

Marijuana Cravings: The most common withdrawal symptom of marijuana is its craving. The person craves marijuana and can't rest until they smoke up.

Mood Swings: The person becomes easily irritable. The moods change and alter quickly, leading from anger, to unhappiness, depression, and euphoria.

Sleeping Difficulties: It becomes hard to fall asleep or stay asleep. Insomnia is common among marijuana users.

Headaches: This is one of the most common symptoms, though some people who withdraw from it may not experience it at all.

It is entirely possible for a person to not experience most of these symptoms, while others may experience all of them. Generally, though, at least three of the symptoms are experienced by the average user, but the extent to which they experience it may vary. Some people only experience mild symptoms while others experience them in their full severity. Experiencing the symptoms to a lesser extent does not mean that you are not dependent on marijuana. Everyone is different and responds to marijuana in different ways.

Chapter 10: Horrors Packed In A Stick Of Cigarette

Smokers always disregard the fact that every stick of cigarette has harmful chemicals as components. Manufacturers put these chemicals there for many purposes such as improvement of flavor, prolongation of shelf life, enhancement of delivery of nicotine to the body, and other related matters.

Current scientific studies have revealed thousands of harmful chemical components in every stick of cigarette. One of the website pages of Tri-County Cessation Center (http://www.tricountycessation.org/tobacofacts/Cigarette-Ingredients.html) shows some of these specific chemicals. The US government requires manufacturers and developers of tobacco products to submit lists of additives they use. Data submission is done on an annual basis and this is how the Health Department is able to summarize risks that smokers have to deal with.

The chemicals listed in the webpage mentioned above are commonly used as food additives. In fact, majority of those were tested to be safe as ingredients to food. However, harmful effects show up after burning these substances. The full extent to which these chemicals harm the body has not been fully uncovered yet. However, there are significant amounts of information already from past studies that can link specific chemical components to major medical conditions like cancer, stroke, blindness, and many others.

Harmful chemicals found in every stick of cigarette can be listed under three big categories. These are as follows:

Cancer Causing (Carcinogens)

Carcinogenic substances are those that can cause cancer. It could also be the factor in the aggravation of an already existing cancer or abnormal tissue growth. Current researches have already identified up to 70 highly active carcinogens in cigarettes. Four of the most harmful are as follows:

Vinyl chloride: This is used in the manufacture of plastics. In case of cigarettes, this is a main ingredient in filters. Aside from liver cancer, it is also responsible for a large number of diseases. These include aggressive forms of allergies, nerve damage, and immunity problems.

BENZENE: This is also present in agricultural pesticides and fuels. Humans have been greatly exposed to this substance for the past couple of decades because of its presence in cigarettes. While a number of medical conditions have been linked to it, the most serious effect to the body is the development of blood cancer or leukemia. Doctors and medical researchers unanimously agree that the chemical plays a vital role in the development of AML and ANLL (Acute Myeloid Leukemia and Acute Non-Lymphocytic Leukemia).

FORMALDEHYDE: Yes, this is the substance used in preserving remains (as in embalming). There are many undergoing researches about the link of formaldehyde to a variety of cancers. However, there are already hard proofs that tie this substance to leukemia and brain cancer. Short-term exposure can produce effects such as eye, throat, and nose irritations, nausea, and skin irritation.

TSNAs: The potency of TSNAs (Tobacco-Specific N-Nitrosamines) as a carcinogenic material in cigarettes is shockingly high.

These are present even in varieties of tobacco products that are smokeless. Even early trials on animals revealed how fast it can lead to the development of tumors. It is directly linked to throat, stomach, and liver cancers.

Poisonous Metals (Heavy Metals)

These include heavy metals used to support life. However, when inhaled or ingested in considerable amounts, it can cause organ or systemic poisoning. It is to be noted that some instances of heavy metal poisoning do not have very visible or aggressive symptoms. An individual might detect its effects when things are already too late or a life-threatening medical condition has already developed.

Examples of identified heavy metal toxins in cigarettes include the following:

CADMIUM: Yes, this is the heavy metal preferred by battery manufacturers at the current times. There are cadmium quantities (safe levels) that can be detected in bodies of humans. Smokers have higher cadmium levels (3-5 times more) in their blood and other body tissues. These levels can cause permanent liver and kidney damage. Inhalation of smoke with cadmium can lead to respiratory allergies and irreversible damage to the lungs.

ARSENIC: This heavy metal has been immortalized in movies and TV shows. The most common household use of arsenic is as ant killer. The progressive ingestion of even low levels of arsenic can kill humans. If high levels of this heavy metal are taken into the body, the toxicity level that will be produced is enough to cause immediate poisoning and death. Lung cancer has been recently tied to arsenic exposure.

The most horrifying discovery about arsenic though is that it has the ability to do damage at the chromosomal level. This means that there are risks of producing sperm or egg cells that are defective. The risk for birth defects, appearance of genetic-linked syndromes, and mutations of cells is very high.

Radioactive Metals: These include isotopes of lead and polonium. When these are accumulated in the body through inhalation, lung cancer is developed. This is the worst effect that these two radioactive metals can produce aside from the usual symptoms of radiation poisoning.

Molecules of lead and polonium are so small that they could penetrate at the cellular level with great ease. This means that such metals can be factors too in the development of other types of cancers.

Common Poisons

Technically, a poison is a substance that can cause physiological distress within a living thing's body. Ultimately, it could cause death. If the list of over 4000 harmful chemical components of cigarettes will be examined, it will be seen that more than half are common poisons. Some of these that people are most likely very familiar with are as follows:

HYDROGEN CYANIDE – Documentary films and TV shows mention this type of chemical being used to kill prisoners in gas chambers during World War 2. Hydrogen cyanide is a colorless and almost odorless chemical, but it has a very high level of toxicity. Inside the body, it causes cellular asphyxiation. It means that the cell's capacity for respiration is cut off. This is the reason why smokers experience shortness of breath and the need to cough.

The human central nervous system (CNS) has high sensitivity to this poison. Even in extremely minute quantities, it could damage nerves, brain cells, and chemical receptors in the brain.

AMMONIA: This chemical compound has a very distinctive smell. It is commonly used in the manufacture of fertilizer and all types of strong cleaners. This is used in cigarettes to improve the quality and speed of delivery of nicotine in the body of smokers.

Ammonia can cause corrosion of the skin and the internal linings of the respiratory system. It can also cause blindness and kill taste and odor receptors. The US Health Department has declared it as a carcinogen just recently. Children, pregnant, and nursing women are most vulnerable to the negative health effects that ammonia could produce.

CARBON MONOXIDE: This has been tagged as the deadly "silent killer". In the US alone, hundreds of cases of carbon monoxide poisoning cases (residential and vehicular) get reported quarterly. Just like cyanide, it is odorless and colorless which makes detection really hard. Inhaling this type of gas can cause headaches, dizziness, vomiting, and loss of consciousness. Long-term exposure to carbon monoxide has been proven to result to heart attack and brain stroke.

The list of horrors that are packed within a stick of cigarette could go on. Ongoing researches about tobacco and other related products are uncovering more information. These are accessible through the information resources available online. The bottom line here is that every stick of cigarette sold out there is as deadly as what anyone could ever imagine.

Chapter 11: Smoking From A Psychological Perspective

Tobacco and Nicotine Addiction

Tobacco is one of the most generally mishandled substances on the planet. It is profoundly addictive. The Centers for Disease Control and Prevention gauges that tobacco causes 6 million deathsTrusted Source for each year. This makes tobacco the leadingTrusted Source reason for preventable demise. Nicotine is the fundamental addictive compound in tobacco. It causes a surge of adrenaline when consumed in the circulatory system or breathed in through tobacco smoke. Nicotine additionally triggers an expansion in dopamine. This is some of the time alluded to as the brain's "upbeat" concoction.

Dopamine animates the territory of the brain related with delight and prize. Like some other medication, utilization of tobacco after some time can cause a physical and mental compulsion. This is likewise valid for smokeless types of tobacco, for example, snuff and biting tobacco.

In 2011, around 70 percentTrusted Source of every single grown-up smoker said they needed to quit smoking. What are the side effects of tobacco and nicotine addiction?

A tobacco fixation is more earnestly to stow away than different addictions. This is to a great extent since tobacco is legitimate, effortlessly got, and can be devoured in broad daylight.

A few people can smoke socially or once in a while, yet others become dependent. A compulsion might be available if the individual:

has withdrawal indications when they attempt to stop (unsteady hands, perspiring, fractiousness, or quick pulse) must smoke or bite after each dinner or after extensive stretches of time without utilizing, for example, after a film or work meeting needs tobacco items to feel "ordinary" or goes to them during times of pressure surrenders exercises or won't go to occasions where smoking or tobacco use isn't permitted keeps on smoking in spite of medical issues. can't quit smoking or biting, regardless of endeavors to stop

What are medicines for tobacco and nicotine enslavement? There are numerous medicines accessible for tobacco compulsion. In any case, this fixation can be hard to oversee. Numerous clients locate that much after nicotine desires have passed, the custom of smoking can prompt a backslide.

There are a few distinctive treatment choices for those fighting a tobacco fixation:

The Patch

The patch is known as a nicotine substitution treatment (NRT). It's a little, wrap like sticker that you apply to your arm or back. The patch conveys low degrees of nicotine to the body. This aides steadily wean the body off it.

Nicotine gum

Another type of NRT, nicotine gum can help individuals who need the oral obsession of smoking or biting. This is normal, as individuals who are stopping smoking may have the desire to place something into their mouths. The gum likewise conveys little dosages of nicotine to enable the you to oversee desires.

Splash or inhaler

Nicotine splashes and inhalers can help by giving low dosages of nicotine without tobacco use. These are sold over the counter and are generally accessible. The shower is breathed in, sending nicotine into the lungs.

Drugs

A few specialists prescribe the utilization of medicine to help with tobacco addictions. Certain antidepressants or hypertension medications may have the option to help oversee yearnings. One drug that is regularly utilized is varenicline (Chantix). A few specialists recommend bupropion (Wellbutrin). This is an upper that is utilized off-mark for smoking end since it can diminish your craving to smoke.

Off-name sedate use implies that a medication that has been endorsed by the FDA for one reason for existing is utilized for an alternate reason that has not been affirmed. Be that as it may, a specialist can in any case utilize the medication for that reason. This is on the grounds that the FDA manages the testing and endorsement of medications, however not how specialists use medications to treat their patients. Thus, your primary care physician can endorse a medication anyway they believe is best for your consideration. Get familiar with off-mark tranquilize use here.

Mental and social medicines:

A few people who use tobacco have accomplishment with strategies, for example,

☐ hypnotherapy
☐ psychological conduct treatment
☐ neuro-etymological programming

These strategies help the client change their musings about habit. They work to adjust sentiments or practices your brain partners with tobacco use. Treatment for a tobacco expansion requires a mix of techniques. Remember that what works for one individual won't really work for another. You should converse with you specialist about what medicines you should attempt.

What is the viewpoint for tobacco and nicotine addiction?

Tobacco addiction can be dealt with appropriate treatment. Addiction on tobacco is like other chronic drug habits in that it's rarely truly restored. As such, it is something that you should manage for a brain-blowing remainder. Tobacco clients will in general have high backslide rates. It's assessed that 75 percent of individuals who quit smoking backslide inside the initial a half year. A more extended treatment period or change in approach may forestall a future backslide.

Exploration has additionally indicated that adjusting way of life propensities, for example, staying away from circumstances where there will be other tobacco clients or executing a positive conduct (like working out) whenever longings start can help improve chances for recuperation.
Step by step instructions to adapt to a smoking backslide »
A tobacco compulsion can have lethal results without treatment. Tobacco use can cause:

☐ malignancies of the lungs, throat, and mouth

☐

coronary illness

☐ stroke

☐ incessant lung sicknesses, for example, emphysema and bronchitis.

Any of these conditions can be deadly. Stopping smoking or tobacco use can essentially lessen the danger of death because of these ailments. Indeed, even once the illness has been analyzed, halting tobacco use can improve treatment endeavors.

Psychological, pharmacological and social factors involved in smoking and smoking cessation.

The regular history of smoking can be displayed as states and factors that impact the progress between these.

Smoking Initiation

Significant variables anticipating initiation in western social orders are: having companions who smoke, having guardians who smoke, low social evaluation, propensity to psychological well-being issues and impulsivity (Action on Smoking and Health, 2015b). Change to day by day smoking follows a profoundly factor design some of the time being quick and once in a while taking quite a while (Schepis and Rao, 2005). Significant variables foreseeing change to standard smoking are: having companions who smoke, frail scholarly direction, low parental help, star smoking mentalities, drinking liquor and low financial status (Action on Smoking and Health, 2015b). Smoking initiation has a 'heritability' (the extent of difference in a trademark that is owing to hereditary as opposed to ecological change) of around 30–half in western social orders (Vink, Willemsen, and Boomsma, 2005). This implies contrasts in hereditary make-up represent practically 50% of the distinction in probability of beginning smoking between people. This doesn't imply that ecological elements don't likewise assume a critical job as is clear from the huge decrease in smoking initiation since the 1970s in numerous western nations.

The heritability of cigarette fixation (as particular from smoking) is roughly 70–80% in western social orders (Vink et al., 2005). Cigarette habit here alludes to the degree to which somebody encounters a solid need to smoke. It is generally filed by a blend of number of cigarettes every day and time from waking to smoking the primary cigarette of the day (Kozlowski, Porter, Orleans, Pope, and Heatherton, 1994). It can likewise be recorded by oneself detailed quality of inclinations to smoke (Fidler, Shahab, and West, 2011). Heritability of cigarette enslavement, as listed by disappointment of endeavors to stop, is higher than the heritability for smoking and for commencement of smoking. This recommends contrasts in hereditary legacy assume a bigger job in having the option to quit smoking than in beginning to smoke.

Cigarette Addiction

Cigarette addiction originates from the way that smoking gives profoundly controllable portions of the medication, nicotine, quickly to the brain in a structure that is open, moderate and acceptable (West, 2009; West and Shiffman, 2016). Nicotine gave all the more gradually, for instance by the nicotine transdermal fix, is considerably less addictive. It is conceivable that at least one mono-amine oxidase inhibitors in tobacco smoke add to, or synergise, the addictive properties of nicotine (Hogg, 2016).

The psychopharmacology of cigarette habit is brain boggling and a long way from completely comprehended. The accompanying sections sum up the current account.

Nicotine takes after the normally happening synapse, acetylcholine, adequately to append itself to a subset of neuronal receptors for this synapse in the brain. These are called 'nicotinic acetylcholine receptors'. At the point when it does this with receptors in the ventral tegmental territory in the midbrain, it causes an expanded pace of terminating of the nerves anticipating forward from that zone to another piece of the brain called the core accumbens. This causes arrival of another synapse called dopamine in the core accumbens. Dopamine discharge and take-up by neurones in the core accumbens is accepted to be key to every addictive conduct. It goes about as a neural 'showing signal' which makes the brain structure a relationship between the current circumstance as saw and the drive to take part in whatever activity promptly went before this discharge. On account of smoking, this makes an inclination to smoke in circumstances where smoking as often as possible happens. These are regularly alluded to as 'prompt driven smoking inclinations' or 'situational longings' (West, 2009; West and Shiffman, 2016). This clarifies why even non-day by day smokers frequently think that its hard to quit smoking through and through. Rehashed ingestion of nicotine from cigarettes makes changes the working of the ventral tegmental zone and core accumbens with the end goal that when brain groupings of nicotine are lower than expected, there is an anomalous low degree of neural movement in these locales. This prompts sentiments of requirement for practices that have in the past reestablished ordinary working, ordinarily smoking. This sentiment of need can be thought of as a sort of 'nicotine hunger', additionally called 'foundation longing for' (West, 2009; West and Shiffman, 2016). This is most likely why time among waking and first cigarette of the day is a helpful indicator of trouble halting smoking (Vangeli, Stapleton, Smit, Borland, and West, 2011). So 'signal driven smoking desires' and 'nicotine hunger' are significant elements adding to smoking conduct and thought to be the essential systems supporting cigarette habit (West, 2009; West and Shiffman, 2016). At the point when smokers keep away from cigarettes, inside a couple of hours a considerable lot of them begin to encounter nicotine withdrawal manifestations. Withdrawal side effects from a medication are brief manifestations that emerge when the medication portion is diminished or use is ended. They emerge from neural adjustment to the nearness of the medication in the focal sensory system. For smoking, the most widely recognized beginning stage indications are: fractiousness, anxiety and troublesome concentrating. Misery and nervousness have likewise been seen in certain smokers. These side effects commonly last 1 to about a month (West, 2009; West and Shiffman, 2016). Following a day or two of halting smoking, numerous smokers experience different side effects: expanded craving, clogging, mouth ulcers, hack, and weight gain. Expanded hunger watches out for keep going for at any rate 3 months; weight gain (averaging around 6 kg) will in general be changeless; different side effects will in general last half a month. The expanded hunger, weight addition and stoppage emerge from end of nicotine admission however the others are most likely identified with different impacts of halting smoking (West, 2009; West and Shiffman,

2016).

Any of the above impacts of restraint may in singular cases advance resumption of smoking after a quit endeavor however factually the affiliation is conflicting and frail; the primary components driving backslide have all the earmarks of being prompt driven smoking inclinations and nicotine hunger (Fidler and West, 2011; West, 2009; West and Shiffman, 2016). Numerous smokers report that smoking encourages them adapt to pressure and builds their capacity to focus. In any case, this seems, by all accounts, to be on the grounds that when they go for a period without smoking they experience nicotine withdrawal side effects that are diminished by smoking. Long haul smokers who stop report lower levels of worry than when they were smoking and no decrease in capacity to think (West, 2009; West and

Shiffman, 2016). It is generally believed that smokers with emotional well-being issues are utilizing cigarettes to 'self-cure' or treat their mental side effects. In any case, the proof demonstrates that neither nicotine nor smoking improves mental side effects, and individuals with genuine emotional wellness issues who quit smoking don't encounter a declining of psychological well- being. Actually a few investigations have discovered an improvement (Royal College of Physicians and Royal College of Psychiatrists, 2013).

Smoking cessation

For most smokers, cessation requires a decided endeavor to stop and afterward adequate purpose in the next many months to defeat what are frequently amazing inclinations to smoke. Elements that anticipate quit endeavors vary from those that foresee the achievement of those endeavors (Vangeli et al., 2011). Around 5% of independent quit endeavors prevail for in any event a half year (Hughes, Keely, and Naud, 2004). Backslide after this point is assessed to be around half over resulting years (Stapleton and West, 2012).

The most well-known self-announced explanations behind smoking are pressure help and delight, with around half of smokers detailing these smoking thought processes. Weight control, supporting focus and mingling are likewise ordinarily refered to (Fidler and West, 2009). Smoking for assumed pressure help, improved fixation, weight control or different capacities has not been seen as identified with endeavors to stop or accomplishment of endeavors to stop (Fidler and West, 2009). Smokers who report getting a charge out of smoking are more averse to attempt to stop yet not less inclined to succeed on the off chance that they do attempt (Fidler and West, 2011). Also, having a positive smoker character (loving being a smoker) predicts doing whatever it takes not to stop, well beyond happiness regarding smoking (Fidler and West, 2009). No unmistakable affiliation has been found between the occasions smokers have attempted to stop previously and their odds of accomplishment whenever they attempt (Vangeli et al., 2011). Nonetheless, having attempted to stop in the previous hardly any months is prescient of disappointment of the following quit endeavor (Zhou et al., 2009). Faith in the damage brought about by smoking is prescient of smokers making quit endeavors however not the accomplishment of those endeavors (Vangeli et al., 2011).

Some clinical examinations have discovered that ladies were more averse to prevail in quit endeavors than men yet huge populace contemplates have discovered no distinction in progress rates between the sexes (Vangeli et al., 2011) so the reality of the situation may prove that ladies who look for help with halting have more noteworthy trouble than men who look for help with halting. Number of cigarettes smoked every day, time among waking and the principal cigarette of the day and appraised quality of inclinations to smoke before a quit endeavor have been found to foresee accomplishment of quit endeavors (Vangeli et al., 2011). Stop endeavors that include continuous decrease are less inclined to prevail than those that include stopping suddenly, significantly in the wake of controlling measurably for proportions of cigarette enslavement, trust in stopping, different strategies used to stop (for example nicotine substitution treatment) and sociodemographic factors (Lindson- Hawley et al., 2016).

Nicotine Addiction

Nicotine reliance happens when you need nicotine and can't quit utilizing it. Nicotine is the compound in tobacco that makes it difficult to stop. Nicotine produces satisfying impacts in your brain, yet these impacts are impermanent. So you go after another cigarette. The more you smoke, the more nicotine you have to feel better. At the point when you attempt to stop, you experience horrendous mental and physical changes. These are manifestations of nicotine withdrawal.

Despite how long you've smoked, halting can improve your wellbeing. It is difficult however you can break your reliance on nicotine. Numerous successful medicines are accessible. Approach your PCP for help.

Symptoms

For certain individuals, utilizing any measure of tobacco can rapidly prompt nicotine reliance. Signs that you might be dependent include:
You can't quit smoking. You've made at least one genuine, yet fruitless, endeavors to stop.
You have withdrawal indications when you attempt to stop. Your endeavors at halting have caused physical and temperament related manifestations, for example, solid yearnings, nervousness, fractiousness, fretfulness, trouble concentrating, discouraged state of brain, dissatisfaction,

outrage, expanded craving, a sleeping disorder, clogging or the runs. You continue smoking in spite of medical issues. Despite the fact that you've created medical issues with your lungs or your heart, you haven't had the option to stop. You surrender social exercises. You may quit going to without smoke eateries or quit associating with family or companions since you can't smoke in these circumstances.

Causes

Nicotine is the concoction in tobacco that keeps you smoking. Nicotine arrives at the brain close to taking a puff. In the brain, nicotine builds the arrival of brain synthetic compounds called synapses, which help manage brain-set and conduct.

Dopamine, one of these synapses, is discharged in the prize focus of the brain and causes sentiments of delight and improved brain-set. The more you smoke, the more nicotine you have to feel better. Nicotine rapidly turns out to be a piece of your day by day schedule and interlaced with your propensities and sentiments. Normal circumstances that trigger the inclination to smoke include:

☐ Drinking espresso or taking breaks at work
☐ Chatting on the telephone
☐ Drinking liquor
☐ Driving your vehicle

☐ Investing energy with companions

To conquer your nicotine reliance, you have to get brainful of your triggers and make an arrangement for managing them.

Risk factors

Any individual who smokes or uses different types of tobacco is in danger of getting needy. Elements that impact who will utilize tobacco include:
Age. A great many people start smoking during youth or the high schooler years. The more youthful you are the point at which you start smoking, the more prominent the possibility that you'll get dependent.
Hereditary qualities. The probability that you will begin smoking and continue smoking might be halfway acquired. Hereditary elements may impact how receptors on the outside of your brain's nerve cells react to high dosages of nicotine conveyed by cigarettes.

Guardians and companions. Youngsters who grow up with guardians who smoke are bound to become smokers. Youngsters with companions who smoke are likewise bound to attempt it. Sadness or other psychological instability. Numerous examinations show a relationship among sorrow and smoking. Individuals who have sadness, schizophrenia, post-horrible pressure issue or different types of psychological maladjustment are bound to be smokers. Substance use. Individuals who misuse liquor and unlawful medications are bound to be smokers.

Complications

Tobacco smoke contains in excess of 60 known malignant growth causing synthetic concoctions and a great many other destructive substances. Indeed "all common" or home grown cigarettes have hurtful synthetic concoctions. You definitely realize that individuals who smoke cigarettes are significantly more prone to create and bite the dust of specific ailments than individuals who don't smoke. Be that as it may, you may not understand exactly what number of various medical issues smoking causes: Lung malignancy and lung malady. Smoking is the main source of lung disease passings. Furthermore, smoking causes lung illnesses, for example, emphysema and incessant bronchitis. Smoking likewise exacerbates asthma.

Different diseases. Smoking expands the danger of numerous sorts of malignant growth, including disease of the mouth, throat (pharynx), throat, larynx, bladder, pancreas, kidney, cervix and a few kinds of leukemia. By and large, smoking causes 30% of all malignant growth passings. Heart and circulatory framework issues. Smoking expands your danger of passing on of heart and vein (cardiovascular) infection, including respiratory failures and strokes. On the off chance that you have heart or vein sickness, for example, cardiovascular breakdown, smoking intensifies your condition. Diabetes. Smoking expands insulin obstruction, which can make way for type 2 diabetes. In the event that you have diabetes, smoking can speed the advancement of confusions, for example, kidney ailment and eye issues.

Eye issues. Smoking can build your danger of genuine eye issues, for example, waterfalls and loss of vision from macular degeneration.

Fruitlessness and barrenness. Smoking expands the danger of diminished fruitfulness in ladies and the danger of feebleness in men.

Intricacies during pregnancy. Moms who smoke while pregnant face a higher danger of preterm conveyance and bringing forth lower birth weight children.

Cold, influenza and different ailments. Smokers are progressively inclined to respiratory diseases, for example, colds, seasonal influenza and bronchitis.

Tooth and gum sickness. Smoking is related with an expanded danger of creating aggravation of the gum and a genuine gum disease that can pulverize the emotionally supportive network for teeth (periodontitis).

Smoking likewise presents wellbeing dangers to everyone around you. Nonsmoking life partners and accomplices of smokers have a higher danger of lung malignancy and coronary illness contrasted and individuals who don't live with a smoker. Youngsters whose guardians smoke are progressively inclined to exacerbating asthma, ear contaminations and colds.

Prevention

The most ideal approach to forestall nicotine reliance is to not utilize tobacco in any case.
The most ideal approach to shield kids from smoking is to not smoke yourself. Exploration has indicated that kids whose guardians don't smoke or who effectively quit smoking are considerably less prone

to take up smoking.

Why nicotine so addictive?

Tobacco use is the top preventable reason for infection and passing in the United States. Cigarettes cause in excess of 480,000 unexpected losses in the United States every year. That is around 1,300 passings consistently. When they begin smoking, individuals as a rule make some hard memories stopping. This is a direct result of the addictive synthetic nicotine, a fundamental fixing in tobacco. In any case, what makes nicotine so addictive?

Brain Training

Expending nicotine—through standard cigarettes or vaping—prompts the arrival of the compound dopamine in the human brain. Similarly as with numerous medications, dopamine prompts or "educates" the brain to rehash a similar conduct, (for example, utilizing tobacco) again and again. This is otherwise called support.

However, here's the trick: The brain gets a dopamine "hit" from nicotine each time an individual takes a puff on a cigarette or breathes in fume from an e-cigarette that contains nicotine.

Endless loop

An average smoker takes at least 10 puffs on every cigarette, so an individual who smokes around one pack (25 cigarettes) day by day gets at any rate 250 "hits" each day. That is a great deal of "instructing" the brain to continue utilizing nicotine. Also, rehashed use expands the danger of fixation.

Regardless of whether an individual devours nicotine through tobacco or vaping, its fortifying impacts may be considerably more unsafe than the client envisions.

This may likewise be the reason youngsters who have a go at vaping (utilizing electronic gadgets like JUUL) frequently change to customary cigarettes—to get increasingly more of the nicotine that the brain presently desires.

Chapter 12: Understanding The Smoking Process

How one would define smoking? In a simple and clear way, it is an addiction to the drug nicotine. After a certain time, it becomes a series of patterns that follow daily routines. Thus, smoking is a psychological condition. The nicotine from cigarettes gives a momentary, and addictive, high. If we eliminate this habitual fix of nicotine, it will cause our body to experience physical withdrawal symptoms and cravings. The nicotine's feel good effect on the brain is the primary reason that makes smokers addicted to it. And it gives us delirious relief from our stress, depression, anxiety, or even boredom.

What is nicotine?

Nicotine is named after Jean Nicot, who introduced this plant to Europe. It is a chemical compound that belongs to the family of nitrogen-based compounds, known as alkaloids. Alkaloids have various psychoactive compounds, such as cocaine, caffeine, and opium.

How does Nicotine affect the brain?

The brain is a complex organ that consists of gray matter and white matter. Gray matter is made up of the cell bodies of neurons and other support cells. White matter is made up of long tracts of axons that link the neurons order to communicate to other brain regions. The brain has billions of neurons, which are networked with each other electrochemically. This nerve stimulation initiates a series of chemical events which in turn creates the electric impulse. What Nicotine does is, it affects the brain activity by altering the working of neurons.

And this is dangerous for the normal functioning of the brain. It acts as a mood enhancer and gives a false feeling of relaxation, which makes it an addictive compound.

Chapter 13: Symptoms Of Nicotine Withdrawal

Nicotine withdrawal happens when the amount of nicotine in your bloodstream starts decreasing. This is the result of reducing the number of cigarettes you smoke, or of completely stopping smoking. Nevertheless, it is more common in people who abruptly stop smoking, compared to those who reduce their consumption slowly.

During the first few weeks of experiencing nicotine withdrawal, different symptoms might start appearing, normally with varying degrees. Some symptoms might be more serious while some might be completely tolerable. Normally, the symptoms will to start disappear after several weeks to a few months.

The most common withdrawal symptoms are:

Headache

Irritability

Anxiety

Drowsiness

Nausea

Difficulty in concentrating

Difficulty in sleeping

Depression

Weight gain or weight loss

Muscle spasm

Craving for cigarette

Other normal symptoms that are not as common as the previously-mentioned ones are:

Diarrhea or constipation

Insomnia

Fatigue

Abnormal hunger

Unusual cravings, especially for sweets

Some of these symptoms might appear all at the same time, but it is also possible that they attack one at a time.

When do the nicotine withdrawal symptoms attack more often?

You can feel them with higher intensity and longer duration at the peak of your emotions, both positive and negative.

Anticipate them so that you can fight the urge consciously at these instances:

Whenever you are stressed out

Whenever you are too worried and nervous

Whenever you feel excited

Whenever you are having so much fun and enjoyment

Whenever you are mad

Surprisingly, clinical findings show that the urge to smoke is not as high as the aforementioned ones when you are sad. The urge is also greatly reduced to almost none when you are mentally active, like while solving a crossword puzzle, writing an essay, or reading a book that stimulates your imagination. Interestingly though, mental activities such as over-thinking, excessive worrying, or catastrophization do not help in preventing smoking urges.

On the contrary, both mental and physical inactivity are strong prerequisites to an urge. This is true even when your body is totally relaxed but your mind remains agitated.

Chapter 14: Self-Hypnosis

Smoking is a psychological habit that has ingrained on your subconscious mind; this is why breaking the habit may require a technique that helps reprogram your subconscious mind.

Most people blame nicotine for their addictions but is nicotine really the problem considering nicotine completely drains out of your system in about 5 days of smoking cessation?

The truth is that you keep smoking because you feel a need to smoke, not because you cannot deal with nicotine withdrawal. It is all in your head and the best way to kick the habit is to focus on the source of the problem. This is where self-hypnosis comes in.

What is Self-Hypnosis?

Self-Hypnosis is a technique that helps you quit smoking by retraining your mind to focus on living a healthier life so you can stop smoking.

Hypnosis is a term used to refer to an altered state of awareness where it seems like you are in a trance or asleep. When you are in that state, you are more willing to "listen to suggestions" because you are relaxed and your level of concentration on the problem at hand is high.

Unlike traditional hypnosis where you would need a professional to get you into a hypnotic state, self-hypnosis requires that you get yourself into a state of hypnosis. When you are in that altered state, you begin to visualize and remind yourself of all the negative effects of smoking as well as how each puff of smoke ravages your body system.

Doing this consistently shall make smoking less desirable to you, which will help keep all the negative consequences of smoking in your mind so that you can make better choices.

Benefits of Self-Hypnosis for Quitting Smoking

The most important benefit is that it helps you successfully quit smoking without having to rely on any replacement therapies. The results of self-hypnosis are usually very quick and long lasting because it increases your willpower. Self-hypnosis is like waking up one day and loathing cigarettes: you cannot stand them anymore and then you quit.

The results can also be gradual and slow but the results are mostly always permanent. If you do not have a lot of money to spend on rehabilitation programs or replacement therapies, this one is free and still easy to use.

Risks and Dangers of the Self-Hypnosis Technique for Quitting Smoking

You may need to dedicate a lot of time to self-hypnosis sessions and this may be a challenge if you are a very busy person. It is also easy to become discouraged if you do not get immediate results.

How to Perform Self-Hypnosis to Quit Smoking

STEP 1: Look for a peaceful and comfortable place where you can practice your sessions for a few minutes without interruptions. You shall need 15-20 minutes to complete a session. Make sure you have enough time so that you do not rush the process.

STEP 2: Sit or lie down depending on whether you have a bed or a chair in your chosen space.

STEP 3: Engage in some breathing exercises to help you relax. Inhale deeply, count from to 5, exhale to a count of 5, and repeat the process until you start feeling calmer and more relaxed.

STEP 4: You should only start hypnosis when you are feeling very calm and relaxed. Think of the waves of the ocean and try to visualize that picture in your mind. Now start imagining that you can see stress and anxiety washing out of your body from the crown of your head to your body. Continue doing this until your muscles relax completely and you start feeling a bit sleepy.

STEP 5: Begin visualizing the smoke from cigarettes getting into your body and ravaging your organs as it goes down.

Visualize how it gets into your brain, blocks oxygen passage, and restricts blood flow. Think of all the potential diseases smoking may cause.

Now imagine living a healthy and smoke free life; visualize it and tell your subconscious mind that this is how you want to feel.

STEP 6: Remain in this state for a few minutes. You can set a timer to help you get out of hypnosis and stop you from falling asleep. When you are ready to come out of hypnosis, count to 10 and wake up slowly.

You are done with your first hypnosis session. Now you just have to repeat this every day until it works for you. You might not get it right in the first try and you may not see the effects the first time but with consistency, you shall soon notice a lessened urge to smoke cigarettes.

Chapter 15: Smoke As Component Of Religious Beliefs

Tobacco and also marijuana were made use of, just like somewhere else on the planet, to verify social relationships, however additionally developed completely brand-new ones. In exactly what is today Congo, a culture called Bena Diemba ("Individuals of Marijuana") was arranged in the late 19th century in Lubuko ("The Land of Relationship").

In modern-day Africa, smoking cigarettes remains in many locations taken into consideration to be modern-day and also an expression of modernity, and also a lot of the solid negative point of views that dominate in the West obtain a lot less focus.".

Marijuana smoking cigarettes prevailed between East prior to the arrival of tobacco, and also was early on a typical social task that focused around the kind of plumbing called a hookah. The water pipes would certainly usually have a number of tubes where greater than someone could possibly smoke each time, or the nozzle would certainly be circulated in the lots of cigarette smoking residences that operated as social centers in significant facilities of Muslim society like Constantinople, Baghdad and also Cairo. Cigarette smoking, specifically after the intro of tobacco, was an important element of Muslim culture as well as society and also ended up being incorporated with essential practices like wedding events, funeral services and also was shared in design, apparel, literary works as well as verse.

In Indonesia, a particular kind of cigarette that includes cloves called kretek was developeded in the very early 1880s as a method of supplying the restorative commercial properties of clove oil, or eugenol, to the lungs. It promptly end up being a prominent coughing solution and also in the very early 20th century kretek started to be marketed as a pre-rolled cigarette (as opposed to being blended as well as rolled by customers). In the 1960s as well as 70s, kretek handled the kind of a nationwide sign, with tax obligation breaks as compared to "white" cigarettes and also the manufacturing started to change from conventional hand-rolling to machine-rolling.

The initial record of a smoking cigarettes Englishman is of a seafarer in Bristol in 1556, seen "releasing smoke from his nostrils". Like tea, coffee and also opium, tobacco was merely one of numerous intoxicants that was initially utilized as a type of medication.

The earliest records of cigarette smoking go back to as very early as 5000 B.C., as well as these documents cover practically every significant social team worldwide. The cigarette smoking of marijuana in India has actually been tape-recorded as early as 4000 B.C.

Since fire damages points entirely, as well as was likewise so required for human survival-- maintaining us cozy, cooking our types of food, and also frightening killers-- it's no surprise that it has such deep spiritual relevance or that it was so fascinating particularly to primitive individuals.

It was smoked in calabash pipes with terra-cotta cigarette smoking bowls, obviously an Ethiopian innovation which was later on shared to eastern, southerly and also main Africa.

International site visitors to the area typically said that smoking cigarettes was greatly prominent amongst Persians; on Ramadan, the Muslim duration of fasting when no types of food was to be consumed while the sunlight was up, amongst the very first point lots of Persians did after sundown was to light their pipelines. Both sexes smoked, but also for ladies it was a personal event appreciated in the privacy of personal houses. In the 19th century Iran was just one of the globe's biggest tobacco merchants as well as the behavior had actually already ended up being something thought about a nationwide Iranian attribute.

Spain and also Portugal were energetic in Central as well as South America, where cigarettes and also stogies were the cigarette smoking devices of selection, as well as their seafarers smoked mainly stogies. Tobacco smoking cigarettes showed up with migrants in the Philippines as well as was presented as early as the 1570s.

By the time Europeans showed up in the Americas in the late 15th century there prevailed usage of tobacco smoking cigarettes as a leisure task. At the receptions of Aztec nobles, the dish would certainly begin by losing consciousness aromatic florals and also cigarette smoking tubes for the supper visitors. At the end of the banquet, which would certainly last all evening, the continuing to be florals, smoking cigarettes tubes as well as types of food would certainly be provided as a type of alms to worn out and also inadequate individuals that had actually been welcomed to witness the get-together, or it would certainly be awarded to the slaves.

Infecting Europe as well as the globe

There is recommendation to tobacco in Persian rhyme dating from prior to 1536. The following trusted eyewitness account of tobacco smoking cigarettes is by a Spanish agent in 1617, yet by now the method was currently deeply engrained in Persian culture. The pipes called qalyan (or hookah) more than likely come from India, yet it remained in Safavid empire Persia that it ended up being a polished cigarette smoking device.

Chapter 16: Withdrawal Symptoms (How To Deal With Them)

When we go about the process of quitting smoking, the first and foremost trouble we face to reach our goal is the withdrawal symptoms and how to deal with them. We can distract ourselves by doing other things, but not only we drain out physically but it is a mental battle too. And we have to win it.

The very common withdrawal symptoms are:

Anger,

Frustration

Irritability

Nicotine cravings

Anxiety

Depression and

Weight gain

Let us now discuss and try to find some solutions to deal with this problem. Firstly we always have to remember at the outset of every step that this is not going to last forever and this is only a temporary feeling. And there is nothing like impossible in my dictionary. You can also experience headaches, dizziness and other symptoms.

The good news is as you go by the process of battling out of this, these symptoms reduces drastically. As you will notice that from the juncture when you started to the date covered after a month, you yourself will feel the difference.

Withdrawal symptoms are something that your body experiences when it is being without the drug called nicotine (the main addictive drug in cigarettes) which causes all the pain and these symptoms. These withdrawal symptoms may vary from person to person, for some it might not be that rigorous or painful, for some, it might feel horrible. And each person might have their own set of withdrawal symptoms other than some general ones. These symptoms depend on a few things like how intensely you smoked or the amount of cigarettes you smoked per day.

Drinking lots of water is beneficial in every aspect for the body, in this case also, it's no different, lots of water flushes out the amount of nicotine quickly from your body, and it also keeps your mouth busy.

Now, as you are preparing yourself to quit smoking or you are already in the process of quitting, you now know the pros and cons of this process, so you must have a solution ready for every possible negative symptoms that attacks you and nullifies your efforts of quitting it, when you find nicotine cravings, be prepared to counter the problem. This way you can be mentally prepared for any pain and any discomfort.

These withdrawal symptoms are not only in your psychology, it's your body's need, the amount of nicotine that your body is used to getting for functioning in your day to day life, so, your cravings might be associated with a lot of things and places, and people or even feelings.

Most smokers say, that whenever they are in stress, or anxiety or in a bad mood or depression, they feel like smoking. Many also say that when they are relaxed and in a good and calm mood they feel like smoking.

Take a deep breath through your nose and exhale slowly through the mouth. Repeat this process 10 times and as often as needed.

Keep your mouth and hand busy, and divert your mind with other thoughts. Work or fiction. Have something healthy to chew on near you, non-addictive and keep your hands engaged by holding pens or coins or anything you may find helpful and suitable, when you are in the process of leaving this bad habit of smoking. You can have dry throat and coughs, and with it you are coughing out phlegm. This is a good sign as your body is trying to cough out the tar and the dirt that has settled down in your lungs. So, don't try and stop it, help your lungs cough it out, until and unless the coughing is unbearable. Try drinking lots of water to fluidity the mucus and make it easier to cough.

Exercises and massage decrease the craving for tobacco. So, whenever you feel the craving for tobacco try them, or you may find yourself irritated; just try relaxing your mind with some relaxing massage or listen to soft music.

Nicotine keeps your mind and body alert, it is a kind of a stimulant so when you try to quit smoking, you find dizziness a problem, it is a good sign; your body is trying to cope without nicotine. So, if possible take a nap and if not, then try to relax your body for a while, don't stretch too far. It's a withdrawal symptoms and it will go with time. You may also experience lack of energy, reason is the same, and your body will need some time to adjust to the new settings. So, give yourself some time.

It may also happen that you have trouble sleeping, in that case nicotine has affected your brain waves and your sleep is also nicotine dependant, and now the brain has to readjust without nicotine, avoid caffeine based drinks like tea coffee or beverages that contain caffeine. This helps to regulate your sleep a lot.

You may also have trouble concentrating, this is nothing but the effect of nicotine in your brain, it is a stimulant and keeps your brain alert, so just help your brain adjust without the stimulant called nicotine, don't not push yourself with extra bit of work for some time and just do what is taxable to the brain. This symptom is not going to last forever.

You might also feel extra hungriness, it's nothing but your brain is getting confused for the nicotine craving with hunger for food and the psychology is also like you have to satisfy yourself with something to fill up your mouth, your heart to satisfy yourself. So, eat healthy meals, balanced diets will suffice and have heart healthy snacks to satisfy the gorge of hunger and the craving to keep your mouth and you busy.

When you can't resist the craving anymore, cause your body and brain wants another hit. Just wait and push yourself. This craving won't last long.

Withdrawal symptoms may be worse at the first day and the first couple of weeks. Some of the minor symptoms stay for 6 months or so, like dizziness, lack of concentration, and depression or even anxiety. Don't bother yourself too much with these symptoms, as they will pass. These symptoms will prove that your body is getting ample amount of oxygen in your lungs instead of nicotine and it is trying to adjust itself and balance with the new environment. So, don't be afraid, neither be bothered. You know in your mind, that you have passed more difficult phases and problems at the outset and still you have managed to quit, so, these niggling bits are not going to frustrate you nor distract you from your goal. You have already achieved what you wanted. A tobacco free life.

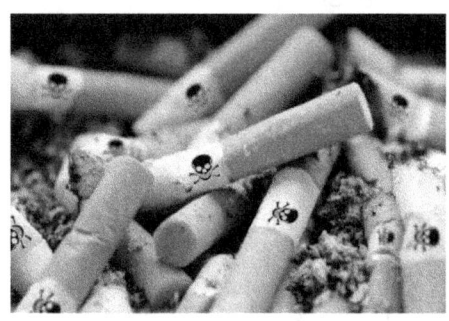

Chapter 17: Plan You Put Down Personally To Stop The Habit Of Smoking

In some case, people who smoke cigarette will just decide to stop by saying "I will not indulge in smoking again" and boom, they will quit the habit instantly, but almost all the smokers need a well crafted plan to keep themselves on the right path. A quitting plan that is good will confront both the challenges that comes with quitting smoking and also the challenges that comes with trying not to go back to smoking after quitting for some time. The plan should also look into your habits associated to smoking and your specific needs.

Ask yourself these questions:

Spend time in thinking about the kind of category you fall to in smoking, which time do you normally feel the urge to light that cigarette stick and the reasons for it. This will give you the enablement to know the therapy, technique and tips that can be very effective for you.

Do you smoke heavily that you can smoke up to one pack each day? Or do you just smoke when in a social gathering or in a party? Is simple nicotine patch okay for you?

Do you have the urge to smoke whenever you visit a certain place, around some set of people, or taking part in some certain activities? Will your craving to smoke increase whenever you finish eating or whenever you're having coffee?

Whenever you're stressed out or feeling down do you considers cigarettes? Or are there other addicted habits that leads to smoking like alcohol addiction, addiction to gambling etc?

Chapter 18: Health

Listing all the diseases caused my smoking, to try to stop you from doing it, is probably not going to be a very effective method. Why? Because you already know that smoking is harmful, right? Turn on the TV or any other media and you are immediately bombarded with various information on smoking. Country after country is joining and initiative to put horrible looking pictures on cigarette boxes. Pictures showing black lungs and other vivid images of human body destruction caused by smoking. Doing so has not shown any noticeable results. Smokers just look the other way or buy protective covers to put over the cigarette box. So much for the scare effect...

Smokers are aware of the risks smoking poses for their health. They know smoking can kill them prematurely, but they still smoke. When it comes to smoking, we are the masters of self-deception. We smoke because we think we are the lucky ones to escape unpunished. We believe there will be some early signs and warnings so we will quit just in time to avoid the bad outcome.

Why then do I have the whole chapter on smoking and health? Because most smokers associate smoking mostly with lung cancer and other lung related diseases, but not much else.

Smoking related diseases

Heart failure

Stroke

Cancers of mouth, nose, throat, lungs, larynx, trachea, esophagus, stomach, pancreas, liver, kidneys, bladder, colon, rectum, cervix, rectal, bone marrow, blood……). The list of cancers is far from complete...

Chronic obstructive pulmonary disease (COPD)

Impotence (if not for anything else men should stop smoking to enjoy in sexual activities even in old age. It is not uncommon for smokers to see impotence developing even as early as mid-30s.)

Asthma and bronchitis

Pneumonia

Diabetes

Gum disease and periodontitis

Losing teeth

Blindness and cataracts

Rheumatoid arthritis

Weakened immune function.

Smoking harms nearly every organ in your body!

Why are cigarettes so dangerous?

It is not the nicotine that does the harm, it is other substances.

Did you know that besides nicotine cigarettes also contain **acetone** (nail polish remover), **ammonia** (used as an agent in toilet cleaners), **arsenic** (used as rat poison), **butane** (also know as lighter gas), **cadmium** (used in rechargeable batteries), **carbon monoxide** (think of car exhaust gases), **formaldehyde**, **lead**, **vinyl chloride**, **insecticides**, **toluene** (used in industrial glue), **naphthalene** (moth killing agent), **methanol** (rocket fuel), **methane** (junkyard gas) **carbon-hydrogen** and even **radioactive polonium 210**. The list is far from complete. Tobacco also contains hundreds of other carcinogenic substances.

Cigarettes contain so many harmful substances that if it were food, you would not think of eating it. Would you ingest something that causes more than ten types of cancer, cardiovascular disease, pulmonary disease and clogged arteries? I don't think there is a person on this planet that would. By inhaling toxic fumes, you are doing something very similar to that.

It is funny how some smokers go all crazy about the BPA in their plastic bottles. They concern themselves about pesticides and all kinds of things, but when it comes to smoking, they do not want to know what the hell they inhale every day.

Is it too late for me?

No matter how old you are and how much you have smoked until now, it is never too late to quit smoking. Studies show that even after a few months after quitting, the risk of developing cardiovascular disease is significantly reduced. So is the risk of getting various cancers. This information can be a double-edged sword. It gives people a false sense of security. They think they can smoke a few more years, quit smoking and just wait a few months and everything will be as if they never smoked. That is far from the reality. Risk of getting a smoking related disease starts dropping immediately after cessation, but does that not mean it drops to zero, not even close to that. It takes almost 20 years for lungs to fully recover, but on the other hand it takes "only" a few years for your heart to return to normal. The bad news is that if you smoke for a long time, some damage done to your lungs is actually irreversible and the amount of damage you cannot reverse or fix increases with time.

If you quit before the age of 40, the amount of damage done is not that significant and likely reversible. If you continue to smoke, more and more tar sticks to your lung cells and it becomes progressively harder for your lungs to function properly. Quitting smoking is very beneficial at any age and it will add years or even decades to your life.

Statistics show that even if you quit smoking at the age of 75, you can still increase your life expectancy by 5 years. But make no mistakes, quitting after 30 years of smoking is much better than doing it after 40 years. The earlier, the better. Do it now!

You never know when you light a cigarette, which will trigger the genetic modification and start the growth of cancer cells. It can happen at the age of 75, but it can also happen at the age of 40 or even sooner. Far too many people wrongfully believe cancer is the disease of the old. For the last forty years, the number of people being diagnosed with cancer at a young age is steadily increasing. So is the number of individuals who suffer a heart attack way before the age of 50. Cancer or cardiovascular disease can strike you at any time. Please, do not think you can smoke for a few more years and then quit without the consequences. Maybe you can, but what if you can't? Are you willing to take that risk? Do you like playing Russian roulette with your life? The odds are against you.

While some people mistakenly believe they have plenty of time to quit smoking, others mistakenly believe that they have already done so much damage that it makes no sense to quit. This thinking is prevalent among long-term smokers and older people. Is adding five years to your life at the age of 75 not reason enough to quit? Is it the same if you die at the age of 75 or live to 80?

If you are currently still in good health, count yourself lucky. You have not yet suffered any smoking-related disease up to this point. Congratulate yourself, but take it seriously. You lucked out and have enough time to quit and prolong your life for many years. Many other people did not get that chance. And once the diagnose is set, there is no way back.

Up to this point, I have been talking mostly about terminal diseases and how much smoking shortens your life. Even more important topic when it comes to quality of life is disability-free years. **Being alive and living is not the same thing.**

While reading smoking related forums, I stumbled across a few posts on emphysema. Those diagnosed with this horrible disease described their suffering in details. Reading those stories can make your hair go up. Some of them wrote how they wish they could die. How they struggle for every breath, not being able to exhale. They feel as if they are suffocation all the time and they have to use a machine to help them exhale the trapped air in their lungs. While they are still alive, is this a life worth living?

Emphysema is only one of the diseases preventing a normal way of living. There are plenty of others. Most of them are preventable; all you have to do is quit smoking. Are you ready?

Think about your future. How your life will look like when you get old. Is your current lifestyle enabling you to grow old and healthy or will you spend the last years of your life wishing you were dead. A disease can be a heavier burden than death.

How do smokers compare to non-smokers regarding various diseases?

The likelihood of a heart failure for smoker is the same as for 15 years older non-smoker! But it does not end there. So is the risk of getting any other smoking related disease. In case you forgot, check the list of all those diseases at the beginning of this chapter.

The risk of getting cancer for the 50 years old smoker is the same as for the 65 years old non-smoker. The difference is very significant. It means that if you currently smoke (which you probably do, why else would you read this book) your body is functioning like that of a 15 years older person than your age. Who wants to live in a body that is almost two decades older than it actually is?

Want more sobering data?

The probability of lung cancer is 20 times higher for smoker, than it is for non-smoker. More than 92% of the cases of lung cancer represent smokers and only 8% represent non-smokers. While lung cancer is not the most prevalent among cancers, it is the most lethal and represents the leading cause of death in EU and USA compared to other cancers. It kills nearly 90% of patients if diagnosed late. Unfortunately, it does not have any noticeable signs in the early stages, so it is usually discovered late.

Smokers, who die from smoking in the middle age, lose on average 22 years of their life. Here we are not even talking disability-free years, in which case the number is even higher.

More than 50% of smokers die because of smoking. If you continue to smoke there is a high chance YOU will die because of it.

In the United States, tobacco use is responsible for nearly one in five deaths; this equals about 480,000 early deaths each year!

Smoking kills nearly 6 million people each year!

Imagine how your life will be easier when you quit. Smokers are constantly under stress. When coughing, you think of lung cancer. You feel the pain in your chest and think of heart failure. I know how smokers think. I thought about cancer a lot. Every cough or chest pain I would think about it and make promises to myself that if I escape without any major disease, I will quit smoking. Even if you do not think about it consciously, you do it unconsciously. Deep inside you know smoking is bad for you, so your mind is under stress. You feel guilty and ashamed of yourself for smoking. All those things are also affecting your health. Researchers are only now discovering how stress can be even more dangerous than smoking. Now imagine yourself, you are a smoker AND under stress. This is a lethal combination.

OK, enough of us, mortals. How about famous people? They can afford much better health care and prevention screening. Does that mean anything? Can medicine protect them from the dangers of smoking? Below is a list of famous people - all died of smoking, mostly way before the age of 60. Keep in mind that the average human lifespan is around 75 years, which means that smoking took anywhere from 20 to 40 years or life from them. The latest to die from smoking related disease this year (2014) is a world known actor Patrick Swayze. He had fame. He had fortune. What good does it make if you cannot enjoy it?

Conclusion

Thank you again for downloading this book!
I hope this book was able to help you to quit smoking or understand what steps to take in order to do so.

The next step is to put into action what you just learned, so you can be a better you and more alive. Also, share this book with anybody who could benefit from this information.

Thank you and good luck!